The Menopause Reset Code

Unlocking Hormonal Harmony for Symptom Alleviation, Weight Mastery, Quality Sleep, and Emotional Wellness Through Peri- and Post-Menopause.

Dr.Maria Martin

Copyright[2023] [Dr.Maria Martin]

Table of content

Introduction

Greetings to everyone! This brings us to the topic of menopause, which affects a lot of women. I would especially like to offer some advice on how to use the Menopause Reset Code to help you get through this stage of life. Take a seat, then, and get ready for some wise advice!

Indeed, menopause is a natural stage of a woman's life. Yes, a lot of physical and emotional changes occur during puberty. It's critical to comprehend menopause and the possible health implications it may have on women. The shift may be considerably simpler with this knowledge. We shall look at the fundamentals of menopause in a lighthearted way in this introduction. We'll concentrate on how crucial it is to approach the issue holistically in order to properly manage its symptoms. Alright, let's get going! Ready to take use of the "Menopause Reset Code" to the hilt and enjoy the benefits that await?

Greetings to everyone! Let's talk about menopause now.

In brief, menopause denotes the conclusion of a woman's reproductive years. The perimenopause, which officially initiates the process, usually occurs in the late 40s or early 50s. Your body experiences hormonal shifts during this period, preparing you for menopause. The three main players in this hormonal orchestra are oestrogen, progesterone, and testosterone.

Why Is the Menopause Significant?

Menopause is more than merely bidding adieu to monthly periods. This hormonal change may result in mood swings, heat flashes, and irregular sleep patterns, among other symptoms. Even while these changes are common, they could be detrimental to a woman's general health.

The Enigmatize Signs of Menopause

A one-size-fits-all strategy to manage menopausal symptoms is not appropriate. It's similar to assembling a puzzle where every piece represents a distinct quality when it comes to a woman's health. Taking into account the mind, body, and spirit entails adopting a holistic approach.

Taking Care of the Reason Not Just the Symptoms

A holistic perspective helps people view menopausal symptoms as linked reactions to hormonal changes rather than as singular occurrences. We go deeper to identify the underlying causes rather than merely addressing specific symptoms. Using a comprehensive approach allows for more practical and long-lasting solutions.

The Menopause Reset Code can be found here.
What is the code for the menopause reset?

To help you navigate the challenges of menopause, consider the Menopause Reset Code as your own customised road map. To assist you in managing your hormones, here is a special blend of dietary advice, lifestyle suggestions, and useful information. This code can help you regain your health and make the most of this period of transformation.

● Reduced Symptoms

Bid farewell to restless nights, volatile moods, and hot flashes. The Menopause Reset Code can alleviate the majority of common menopausal symptoms, restoring your autonomy over your day-to-day activities.

• Control of Weight

Learn how to effectively control your weight both during and after menopause. Put fad diets and fast solutions aside; this is about long-term strategies to boost your energy and health.

• Restful Nights

Goodbye to insomniac nights. You can ensure that you awaken with a refreshed sense of energy and vitality by heeding the practical instructions provided in The Menopause Reset Code.

• Emotional and psychological health

Remain composed while you ride the emotional rollercoaster. With the help of the code, you may improve your mental health, boost your resilience, and adopt an optimistic outlook.

An overview of what will happen next
The Menopause Reset Code will provide fresh perspectives and doable actions for each chapter as we set out on this journey together. Hormonal balance and much more will be covered, along with a host of other issues like controlling weight, getting enough sleep, maintaining mental stability, and embracing change.

Are you prepared to enter the Menopause Reset Code and face this transformative phase with confidence? Come learn the keys to hormone balance, symptom relief, and living a vibrant, healthful life!

Chapter 1: Menopausal Transition

Menopause is a normal stage in a woman's life. It's a time when her body undergoes changes, particularly in the hormones that influence how she feels and functions. Let's look at this trip through the lens of perimenopause, the period preceding menopause, and see why keeping these hormones in balance is so important for feeling good overall.

Managing Hormonal Shifts

When we talk about hormones, we're referring to the messengers in the body that control numerous functions. These hormones begin to fluctuate during perimenopause, which is like the warm-up period before menopause.

Oestrogen, progesterone, and testosterone work as a team, and when they are out of sync, a woman's mood suffers.

Why Do Hormonal Shifts Matter?

Consider hormones to be traffic lights. Everything runs nicely when they are in balance. However, during perimenopause, it's as if the traffic lights change abruptly, producing some traffic backups. This can cause symptoms such as heat flashes, mood fluctuations, and sleep problems.

Understanding Hormonal Balance's Importance

Consider the body to be a seesaw. For the seesaw to keep level, oestrogen, progesterone, and testosterone must be balanced. If one hormone is too high or too low, the seesaw will tip, resulting in symptoms. This hormonal balance impacts not just the body, but also how a woman thinks and feels.

Taking Initiative

Understanding the changes is the first step, but what follows is critical—taking action to successfully navigate this transition. Let's look at ways to accept the physical and emotional changes that come with menopause.

Accepting Change

Menopause is a fresh beginning, not an end. It's like starting a new school or playing a new game. The first step is to adopt an optimistic attitude. Instead of seeing it as something to be afraid of, consider it an opportunity for growth and progress.

Developing a Positive Attitude

Consider this: a garden. Menopause is similar to growing new seeds. With the appropriate attitude, those seeds can blossom into lovely blooms. Encouragement, such as "I can handle this," and "This is a natural part of life," can make a significant difference.

Adaptation Techniques for Physical and Emotional Changes

Adapting to menopause needs work, much like learning to ride a bike or play a new game. Let's look at some easy ways for dealing with both physical and emotional changes.

Physical Modifications

Exercise isn't about running marathons; it's about finding activities you enjoy, such as walking, dancing, or even gardening.

Healthy Eating: Consider your body to be an automobile. It requires the proper fuel to run smoothly. Consuming fruits, veggies, and whole grains gives your body the energy it requires.

Emotional Shifts

Express Yourself: Expressing your thoughts, like colouring in a colouring book, can be beneficial. Talk to friends, keep a journal, or seek out creative outlets.

Mindfulness is similar to stopping to smell the flowers throughout a hectic day. Mindfulness exercises, such as deep breathing or moderate yoga, can promote relaxation.

Steps to Take to Prepare for the Transition

Now, let's get down to business—practical things you can take right now to make this shift go more smoothly.

● **Build a Support System:**

Share your emotions with friends and family. It's like having teammates rooting for you.

● Prepare Yourself:

Power comes from knowledge. Learn about menopause so you can be prepared.

● Make self-care a priority:

Consider yourself a superhero. Get enough sleep, eat healthily, and devote time to things that you enjoy.

● Small victories should be celebrated:

Every day is an improvement. Celebrate small achievements, such as trying a new healthy recipe or going for a 10-minute stroll.

● Keep an Open Mind:

Approach this voyage with a sense of adventure, as if you were exploring a new track. Every day is a fresh adventure to be had.

To summarise, the menopausal transition is a journey rather than a destination. This transition may be a time of growth and empowerment if you navigate hormonal shifts, recognize their significance, and take constructive activities. Accept the changes, adapt with a good attitude, and take actionable actions to personalise this trip. Remember that you are not alone on this journey.

Chapter 2:Blueprint for Hormonal Harmony Encodement

Hormones act in our bodies as tiny messengers. They influence how we feel and function. Let's take a closer look at three important hormones: oestrogen, progesterone, and testosterone, and see how they interact with one another.

Oestrogen: An Overview

Consider oestrogen to be your body's superpower. It promotes bone health, skin health, and even mood.

Progesterone:

Progesterone is a soothing companion. It aids in oestrogen balance and promotes a healthy menstrual cycle.

Testosterone:

Women have testosterone, too! It increases energy, promotes muscle health, and preserves vitality.

Hormonal Changes and Menopausal Symptoms

Consider hormones to be a crew on a boat. Everything is OK if the boat is sailing nicely. However, the hormonal boat might rock during menopause, resulting in symptoms such as hot flashes, mood swings, and changes in sleep habits. Understanding these variations is like predicting when the seas will get stormy.

Act of Balancing

Now that we've gotten a glimpse into the world of hormones, let's speak about how to keep them in balance. It's like ensuring that all of the instruments in a band perform in unison. We'll look at natural approaches to balance, such as what you eat and how you live, as well as some herbal remedies.

Natural Hormone Balance Treatments Hormonal Balance Nutritional Interventions:

Eating the correct meals is like providing your hormones with a nutritious meal. Fruits, veggies, and whole grains are high in vitamins and minerals and can help keep your hormones in balance.

Changes in Lifestyle to Promote Hormonal Balance:

Lifestyle is similar to the beat of a song. Regular exercise, enough rest, and stress management help to keep your hormones in tune.

Balanced Herbal Remedies and Supplements:

Consider herbs and supplements to be the band's backup singers. They are willing to assist when necessary. Black cohosh and evening primrose oil are examples.

Let's take it a step further:

Hormonal Balance Nutritional Interventions:

• Veggies and fruits:

Consuming colourful fruits and vegetables provides your body with a rainbow of nutrients. They are rich in vitamins and antioxidants, which help to maintain hormonal equilibrium.

• Complete Grains:

Brown rice and quinoa, for example, are like the strong foundation of a pyramid. They give consistent energy and fibre, both of which are essential for hormonal health.

Fats That Are Good for You:

Consider avocados and nuts to be the nice guys in your hormonal drama. They help to produce hormones and keep everything functioning smoothly.

Changes in Lifestyle to Promote Hormonal Balance:

● **Regular Physical Activity**:

Exercise is a hormonal dance. It keeps them on track and lifts your spirits. Try activities you like, such as walking, dancing, or sports.

● **Good Sleep:**

Sleep acts as a hormonal reset button. Each night, aim for 7-9 hours of high-quality sleep.

Create a relaxing nighttime routine to aid in relaxation.

• Stress Control:

Stress is a storm that can upset hormonal balance. Find things that can help you relax your thoughts, such as deep breathing, meditation, or spending time outside.

Balanced Herbal Remedies and Supplements:

• The herb black cohosh

Menopausal symptoms are soothed by black cohosh. This herbal medicine has helped some women deal with hot flashes and mood swings.

• Evening Primrose Oil (Evening Primrose Oil):

Evening primrose oil is a backstage access to hormonal harmony. It has gamma-linolenic acid, which may help alleviate breast pain and other symptoms.

Finally, deciphering hormones and attaining hormonal balance is like leading a symphony. Understanding the roles of oestrogen, progesterone, and testosterone, as well as using natural measures such as nutrition, lifestyle, and herbal support, can help you build a beautiful tune for your overall well-being. It's not about complex answers; it's about making simple, everyday decisions that keep your hormonal orchestra in tune.

Chapter 3: Strategies for Symptom Relief

Unravelling Menopausal Symptoms

Menopause brings about changes, and recognizing how they can impact you is the first step toward obtaining relief. Let's look at some common symptoms, keeping in mind that each woman's experience is unique.

Identifying Common Symptoms Hot Flashes:

Hot flashes are brief bursts of heat that might cause flushing. Consider your body experiencing a brief, unexpected heatwave.

- **Mood Swings:**

Mood swings are similar to emotional rollercoasters. Some days may be joyous, while others may be frustrating or sad.

• Insomnia:

Insomnia occurs when sleep decides to play hide-and-seek. The Sandman may appear to be on vacation.

And there's more:

Other symptoms may include changes in libido, joint pain, or amnesia. It's as if your body is sending you messages to let you know it's adjusting.

Individualised Menopausal Symptoms

Just as no two snowflakes are alike, no two women experience menopause in the same manner. Your path is unique, and recognizing your specific symptoms is critical to finding the proper answers.

Alternative Treatments

Now that we've identified the most prevalent symptoms, let's look into natural and holistic solutions that go beyond merely treating the surface. Consider it as providing your body with a whole wellness kit.

Mind-Body Techniques for Symptom Relief:

Meditation is like a mini-vacation for your mind. It helps to quiet the whirlwind of thoughts and relieves tension.

Yoga is a peaceful dance for your body. It mixes movement and awareness to promote relaxation.

Alternative Therapies:

- **Acupuncture**: Acupuncture is similar to tapping into your body's natural energy flow. It uses tiny needles to relieve problems.

- **Massage**: Massage is like a calming song for your muscles. It relieves tension and promotes relaxation.

Personalized Approaches to Symptom Management:

Consider a toolbox full of solutions designed specifically for you. It could include a combination of lifestyle changes, dietary alterations, and particular techniques that are tailored to your personal needs.

Let's break it down further:

Mind-Body Techniques:

- **Meditation**:

Find a quiet place, close your eyes, and take calm, deep breaths. Imagine your anxieties floating away like leaves in a peaceful stream.

- **Yoga**:

Begin with easy positions. Stretch softly, breathe deeply, and let the tranquil rhythm of yoga relax both body and mind.

Acupuncture is one of the alternative therapies.

Consider small needles to be your aides. They can target specific areas, improving balance and easing discomfort.

● **Massage**:

A massage is like a warm hug for your muscles. It increases blood flow and relieves stress, bringing comfort.

Personalized Approaches to Symptom Management:

● **Changes in Habits:**

Determine the factors that aggravate symptoms. If stress is the problem, consider incorporating relaxation techniques into your regular practice.

● **Dietary Changes:**
Some meals may worsen symptoms. Experiment with your diet, concentrating on nutritious foods and being hydrated.

Practices That Are Right For You:
Investigate what gives you delight. These personalised habits, whether gardening, drawing, or spending time in nature, contribute to your well-being.

To summarise, recognizing the particular language your body speaks is essential for deciphering menopausal symptoms. You can construct a tailored path to symptom treatment by recognizing common symptoms and researching holistic solutions such as mind-body practices, alternative therapies, and individualised approaches. Remember, it's not just about addressing the surface; it's about embracing a holistic approach that nurtures your mind, body, and soul on this transformational journey.

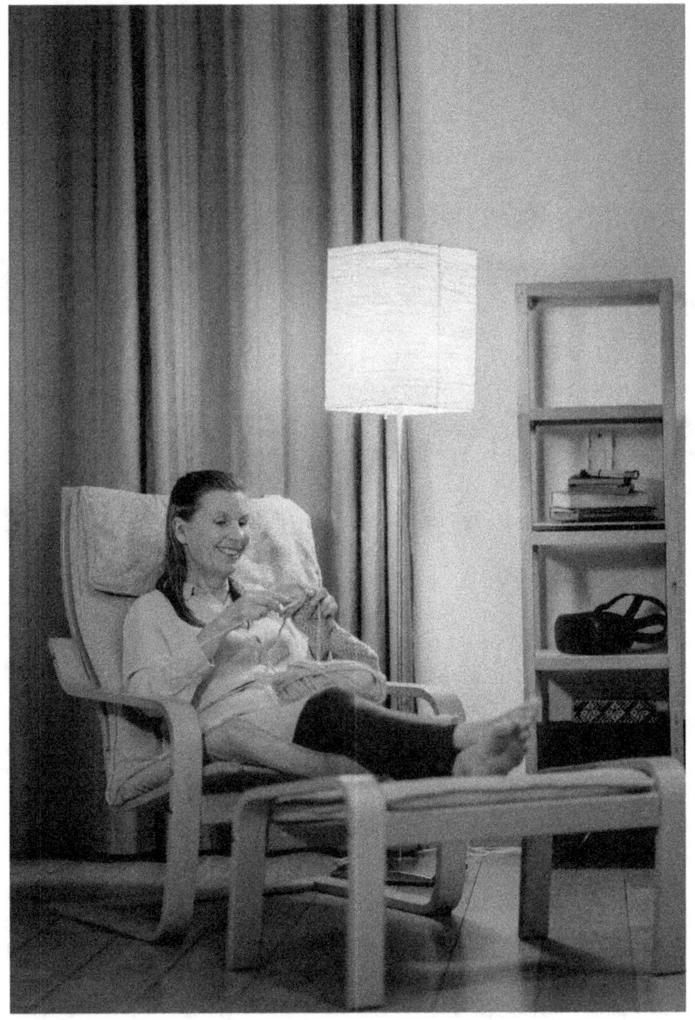

Chapter 4: Weight Control

Menopause and Weight

Let's look at how menopause affects your weight. Understanding the backstage of a magic show is similar—there's more to it than meets the eye.

Understanding Metabolic Shifts:

Metabolic shifts are analogous to the changing of gears in your body's engine. Your body may burn calories in a different way during menopause.

Hormonal Weight Influence:

Hormones behave as conductors in an orchestra. Oestrogen and other hormone fluctuations can have an impact on how your body stores and uses energy.

Differentiating Between Muscle Gain and Fat Gain

Consider your body to be a structure. It's critical to understand whether you're gaining weight (fat growth) or losing muscle mass (muscle loss). Let's simplify everything.

Weight Control Made Simple

Now that we've established the link, let's move on to practical steps—real-world behaviours that will help you manage your weight throughout and after menopause.

Customised Exercise Routines:

In the story of weight loss, exercise is a superhero. Make your own routines, such as walking, swimming, or dancing. Discover what gives you joy.

Nutritional Plans:

Consider your body a garden. Feed it a vibrant assortment of fruits, veggies, and nutritious grains. It's not about following a rigorous diet, but about making healthful choices.

Changes in Way of Life:

The setting of a play is similar to lifestyle. Rest healthily, reduce stress, and devote time to things that you enjoy. It is all about long-term, sustainable transformations.

Let's take it a step further:

Exercise Programs:

• Walking:

Go for a walk around your neighbourhood. It's simple, entertaining, and keeps your body moving.

• Swimming :

Dive into the swimming pool. Swimming is easy on the joints and provides a terrific total-body workout.

● **Dancing**:

Put on your favourite music and get ready to dance. It's more than just a workout; it's pure entertainment.

Nutritional Plans:

● **Plate of Colors**:

Make a rainbow of colours on your plate. Different fruits and vegetables have a wide range of nutrients that your body requires.

● **Complete Grain:**

Brown rice and whole wheat bread are examples of entire grains. They satisfy your hunger and provide long-lasting energy.

● **Hydration:**

Keep hydrated. It's like giving your body a breather.

Changes in Way of Life:

● **Good Sleep**:

Each night, try to get 7-9 hours of sleep. It's your body's method of getting ready for the next day.

● **Stress Control:**

Find relaxing hobbies, such as reading, listening to music, or taking a warm bath.

● **Happy Activities:**

Do things that make you happy, such as gardening, drawing, or spending time with family and friends.

Finally, the menopause-weight relationship is like a puzzle with usable pieces. Recognize the changes, distinguish between fat gain and muscle loss, and arm yourself with targeted exercise, nutrition, and lifestyle modifications. It's not about following rigid rules; it's about finding delight in taking care of oneself during this transitional period.

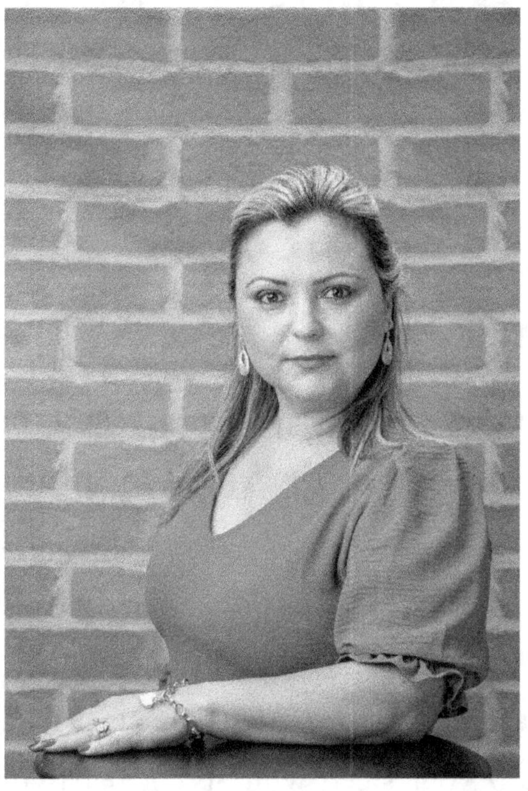

Chapter 5: Quality Sleep Solutions

Sleep Disruptions During Menopause

Let's talk about sleep during menopause. It's like discovering a new universe where nocturnal escapades aren't always as romantic as we'd like them to be.

Examining Sleep Issues Insomnia:

Insomnia occurs when sleep becomes a game of hide and seek. You want it, yet it can be difficult to obtain.

● **Night Sweats:**

Night sweats are like unexpected summer rain. They disturb your sleep with abrupt bursts of heat.

● Sleep Architecture Changes:

Sleep architecture alterations are similar to remodelling your sleep structure. The patterns shift, affecting how deep and peaceful your sleep is.

The Effect of Sleep Deprivation on Overall Well-Being

Consider sleep to be the superhero cape for your well-being. When it's not at its best, everything else may feel a little shaky.

Making a Restful Night

Now, let's get started on making a night that feels like a warm, comfortable, and welcome blanket.

Establishing a Sleep-Friendly Environment:

Your bedroom is a haven for excellent sleep. Make it dark, quiet, and cool. It's your personal sleeping haven.

Relaxation Techniques for Better Sleep Quality:
Relaxation is like a soft lullaby for your thoughts. Before bedtime, try deep breathing, easy stretches, or even gentle music.

Melatonin and Other Sleep Supplements:
Melatonin is like the sandman's assistant. It tells your body that it's time to unwind. Supplements can occasionally provide that extra nudge.
Let's break it down further:

Creating a Sleep-Friendly Environment:
Darkness:

Block out light with curtains or an eye mask. It's like telling your brain, "It's time for darkness now."

Quietness:

Earplugs or calming sounds can help you create a tranquil cocoon. It's like turning down the volume on the world.

Temperature: cool

Keep your room cool. It's easy to snuggle into your covers when the temperature is exactly right.

Relaxation Techniques for Better Sleep Quality:

● **Deep Breathing**:

Slowly inhale and exhale. Repeat. It's like a mental vacation.

- **Simple Stretches:**

Stretch your arms and legs gently. It's like giving your body a gentle wakeup call to prepare for rest.

- **Soft Music:**

Listen to soothing music. It's like a lullaby for your ears, signalling that it's time to unwind.

Melatonin and Other Sleep Supplements:

Melatonin:

Consider melatonin pills, but always consult a parent or doctor first. It's like a small helper informing your body it's time to sleep.

- **Herbal Teas:**

Some teas, such as chamomile, can be calming. It's like drinking warmth and calm.

- **Magnesium Supplements:**

Magnesium can occasionally help with relaxation. Consider it a slight nudge to your muscles to unwind.

Finally, quality sleep is like a treasure vault for total well-being. Investigate the difficulties, establish a sleep-friendly environment, practice relaxing techniques, and think about gentle supplements. It's not just about going to bed; it's about creating a restful night that sets the tone for a vibrant and enthusiastic morning.

Chapter 6: Emotional Wellness Strategies

Managing the Emotional Rollercoaster

Let's discuss feelings throughout menopause. It's like riding a rollercoaster, and we're learning out how to embrace the twists and turns.

Menopausal Emotional Challenges Mood

- **Swings**:

Mood swings are like unexpected weather changes in your emotions. You may be bright one minute and then have a storm the next.

- **Irritability**:

Irritability occurs when little irritations become major irritants. It's like having a grouchy cloud about.

● **Emotions are heightened:**

Emotions may be loud. It's like cranking up the volume on sensations, making them more intense.

Hormonal Fluctuations' Psychological Impact

Consider hormones to be the conductors of your emotional symphony. Everything runs nicely when they are in sync. However, during menopause, the orchestra may play a little off-key.

Emotional Resilience Development

Now, let's look at how to be the superhero of your own emotions, developing resilience to deal with the ups and downs.

Mind-Body Practices for Emotional Well-Being Cognitive-Behavioral Strategies for Emotional Resilience:
Cognitive-behavioural methods are like tools in a superhero's arsenal. They assist you in changing negative thinking and managing your emotions.

Expressive Arts and Journaling for Emotional Release:
Expressive arts are a creative outlet for your emotions. Drawing, writing, or any other kind of art may be like opening a doorway allowing emotions to flow through.

Creating a Helpful Social Network:

A helpful social network is similar to a squad of sidekicks. Friends and relatives give support and understanding.

Let's break it down further:

Cognitive-Behavioral Strategies for Emotional Resilience:

•Positive Self-Talk:

Talk to yourself like a buddy. It's like having a cheerleader in your head telling you that you're powerful.

• Problem-Solving Capabilities:

Break down large issues into little stages. It's like putting together a puzzle—one piece at a time.

• Mindfulness:

Be in the moment. It's like clicking the stop button to appreciate what's going on right now.

Expressive Arts and Journaling for Emotional Release:

- **Drawing**:

Draw what you are feeling. It's similar to making a visual tale for your feelings.

- **Writing**:

Keep a journal. It's like pouring out your emotions into paper and giving them a home.

- **Dancing or singing**:

Move your body or sing along to music. It's like allowing the beat to say what words cannot.

Creating a Helpful Social Network:

- **Maintain Regular Contact:**

Talk to your friends or relatives. It's like sharing your mental load, so it doesn't seem so heavy.

● **Join Groups or Clubs**:

Being a member of a group is like having a circle of understanding. You share your experiences and help each other.

● **Seek Assistance**:

Don't be afraid to seek assistance. It's like holding out your hand when you need someone to grasp it.

To summarise, emotional wellbeing is similar to tending to a garden of sentiments. Navigate the obstacles, grow resilience via mind-body activities, and create a supporting network. Remember that emotions are like waves that come and go. By using these tactics, you're not simply riding the emotional rollercoaster; you're driving it in a more pleasurable direction.

Chapter 7:Peri-Menopause Nutritional Needs

Understanding what your body requires throughout perimenopause is similar to having a tailored guidebook for this stage of your life.

Changing Nutritional Needs

● **Addressing Nutrient Deficiencies:**

Nutrient shortages are analogous to missing jigsaw parts. For total well-being, we must identify and fill these deficiencies.

● **The Importance of a Well-Balanced Diet**:

A well-balanced diet is analogous to a superhero outfit. It delivers the necessary nutrients to counteract menopausal symptoms and keep you feeling powerful.

Menopause Superfoods

Let's speak about foods that can be your allies during perimenopause, like having a squad of superheroes on your plate.

• Phytoestrogens and antioxidant-rich foods for symptom relief:

Phytoestrogens and antioxidants act as shields and armour. They protect your body against the effects of perimenopause.

• Essential vitamins and minerals:

Essential vitamins and minerals are like the items in your superhero utility belt. They play critical functions in maintaining your health throughout menopause.

•Personalized Nutrition Plans:

Consider a tailored nutrition plan as your one-of-a-kind approach. It takes into account your tastes and requirements, guaranteeing that you can keep to the plan.

Let's break it down further:

Including Phytoestrogens and Antioxidants:

• Phytoestrogens:

These are like helpful aides that imitate oestrogen in your body. They may be found in foods including soy, flaxseeds, and whole grains.

• Antioxidants:

Antioxidants act as guardians, safeguarding your cells. Berries, nuts, and bright veggies are all high in antioxidants.

Essential vitamins and minerals:

• Vitamin D:

Consider vitamin D to be the "sunshine vitamin." It is necessary for bone health. It's found in fatty fish, eggs, and fortified meals.

● **Calcium**:

Calcium acts as the building blocks for strong bones. It's found in dairy, leafy greens, and fortified plant-based milk.

● **Magnesium**:

Magnesium acts as a muscle relaxant. It's found in nuts, seeds, and whole grains.

Personalized Nutrition Plans:

● **Identify Preferences:**

Consider the meals you prefer. It's similar to adapting your strategy to your preferences.

● **Include Variety:**

A diverse diet promotes a balance of nutrients. It's like recruiting various superheroes to join your squad.

● **Listen to Your Body:**

Pay attention to how your body reacts to various meals. It's like studying the language of your body.

Finally, perimenopause nutrition is about fuelling your body with the proper nutrients. Address vitamin shortages, adopt a balanced diet, and make power foods your allies. Include phytoestrogens, antioxidants, and vital vitamins and minerals. With a tailored nutrition plan, you're not simply eating; you're developing a strategy to maintain your health throughout this transitional period.

Chapter 8: Long-Term Health Benefits of Post-Menopausal Fitness Exercise

Let's speak about how to keep active after menopause—it's like giving your body a superhero exercise in the long term.

Exercise and Postmenopausal Bone Health:

Exercise is like a bone superhero. It maintains them healthy and prevents problems like osteoporosis.

• Cardiovascular Advantages

Cardio exercise, such as walking or dancing, acts as a heart superhero. It maintains your ticker health and robustness.

● Mood Elevation:

Exercise is a natural mood enhancer. It causes you to feel joyful by releasing pleasant chemicals.

Postmenopausal Fitness Routines

Your fitness plan, like superheroes' outfits, should be suited to your postmenopausal demands.

Practices of Holistic Fitness

Let's look at several activities that might help you feel better overall, kind of like a superhero squad.

Yoga, Strength Training, and Cardio for Postmenopausal Women

Consider your fitness routine to be a one-of-a-kind attire. It is ideal for you, taking into account your fitness level and tastes.

Mindfulness Integration

Mindfulness is like a workout buddy. It allows you to remain in the present moment by linking your mind and body.

Monitoring and Adaptation:

Progress tracking is similar to maintaining a journal of your heroic exploits. It allows you to monitor how far you've progressed and change your plans as necessary.

Let's take it a step further:

Creating Your Own Workout Routine:

Begin Slowly:

Begin with activities that you find enjoyable. It's like slipping into a cosy superhero costume.

Include a variety of items:

Mix up your activities by going for a stroll, dancing, or taking a fitness class. It's like having a varied group of superheroes on your squad.

Take Notice of Your Body:

Pay attention to how you feel in your body. It's like talking to your body and making sure it's comfy and pleased.

Mindfulness Integration

Take a deep breath:

During exercising, keep your attention on your breathing. It's as if you're welcoming tranquillity into your exercise.

Take Advantage of the Situation:

Take note of the movement. It's similar to appreciating every frame of a superhero film.

Be Gentle with Yourself:

It's OK if an exercise is difficult. It's a little like giving oneself a pep talk.

Monitoring and Adaptation:

Establish Achievable Objectives:

Aim for modest wins. It's similar to accumulating superhero badges along the road.

Milestones should be celebrated:

Celebrate your successes. It's similar to arranging a superhero party for yourself.

Adapt as Required:

Adapt your strategy if something isn't working. It's like changing the direction of a superhero's trip.

Finally, post-menopause exercise is about maintaining your superhero body. Exercise improves bone health, heart health, and mood. Make exercise a comprehensive discipline by tailoring your regimen, including yoga, weight training, and cardio. Make your own goals, include mindfulness, and measure your progress—this isn't just exercise; it's a superhero training program for a flourishing post-menopausal existence.

Chapter 9:Menopause Brain Health

Cognitive Transitions and Difficulties

Let's talk about the brain during menopause—it's like a superhero headquarters going through some changes, and we're trying to figure out how to keep it in top shape.

Memory Gaps and Cognitive Shifts:
Memory lapses are like tiny flashes on your superhero radar. Things may slip away at times.

Cognitive Impairment:
Cognitive fog settles in like mist. It can cause your thoughts to become foggy.

Issues with concentration:

Concentration problems are similar to trying to focus in a noisy environment. It requires a little more effort.

Hormonal Relationship and Brain Health

Consider hormones to be messengers that send messages to the brain. During menopause, the messaging system receives a superhero makeover.

Brain Boosting Techniques

Now, let's look at ways to strengthen your brain's superhero abilities, keeping it sharp and ready for action.

Cognitive Exercises and Lifestyle Habits for Cognitive Well-being

Cognitive exercises are like brain training sessions. They improve memory and focus, allowing you to keep your mental muscles strong.

• **Brain Nutrition**:

Nutrition serves as brain fuel. Foods high in omega-3 fatty acids, antioxidants, and vitamins help it perform its superhuman duties.

•**Stress Control**:

Stress management functions as a protective shield for your brain. It promotes cognitive resilience, which helps keep your superhero headquarters calm.

Let's take it a step further:

Mental Workouts:

• **Memory Activities**:

Take part in memory games. It's similar to doing push-ups for your brain to keep it flexible.

- **Crossword puzzles and crossword puzzles:**
Complete crossword puzzles and puzzles. It's like a mental obstacle course that will test your brain in new and exciting ways.

- **Discover something new:**
Learn a new skill or hobby. It's like bestowing a new superhero power on your brain.

Brain Nutrition:

- **Fatty acids omega-3:**
Include foods like fish and nuts in your diet. They're like brain food.

Foods High in Antioxidants

Berries and dark leafy greens, disguised as superheroes, fight off harmful molecules in your brain.

Minerals and vitamins

Consume a diverse range of fruits and vegetables. They work together as a nutrient-rich team to support the health of your brain.

Deep Breathing for Stress Reduction:

Deep breathing is recommended. It functions as a calming technique, assisting your brain in remaining focused.

Breaks on a regular basis:

Take breaks as necessary. It's the equivalent of pressing the reload button on your superhero headquarters.

Nature Trails:

Spend time outside. It's like a mental retreat, providing moments of calm.

Finally, brain health during menopause is about assisting your superhero command centre. Understanding cognitive shifts, engaging in mental exercises, prioritising brain-friendly nutrition, and managing stress are all important. It is not about avoiding changes, but about ensuring that your brain remains a vibrant superhero throughout your life's journey.

Chapter 10: Revitalization of Sexual Health

Navigating Sexual Health Transitions

Understanding changes in how you feel and connect intimately is similar to embarking on a new adventure in your superhero story.

Menopause Sexual Difficulties Vaginal Dryness:

Vaginal dryness is similar to a superhero cape that requires special care. It's common and can interfere with intimacy.

Libido reduction:

Reduced libido is analogous to pressing the pause button. It's not the end; it's just a change in tempo.

Issues with Intimacy:

Intimacy issues are similar to communication breakdowns. They can be overcome with patience and understanding.

Rediscovering Intimacy Consider rediscovering intimacy to be like unearthing a treasure chest of emotions and connection—similar to discovering a new way for your superhero team to collaborate.

Sexual Health: A Holistic Approach

Let's look at holistic ways to keep the flames of intimacy burning bright, such as boosting your superhero relationship.

Sexual Vitality Exercises for the Pelvic Floor

- **Pelvic Floor Workouts**:

Pelvic floor exercises are similar to strength training for the muscles in your intimate area. They increase flexibility and sensation.

•Emotional connection and communication: Communication is like the superheroes' secret language. To strengthen the emotional bond, express your emotions, fears, and desires.

• Pleasure-Focused Practices: Pleasure-oriented practices are analogous to adding some fun gadgets to your superhero toolkit. Sensual messages, exploration, and mutual understanding could be among them.
Let's take it a step further:

Pelvic Floor Workouts:
• Kegels:
Squeeze and then relax the pelvic muscles. It's like putting them through a workout to keep them in shape.

- **Exercising the Bridge:**

Raise your hips to the sky. It feels like a pelvic floor stretch.

- **Squatting:**

Squats are a good exercise. It's similar to a full-body exercise for your pelvic muscles. Emotional connection and communication:

- **Express Your Emotions:**

Express yourself freely. It's the equivalent of connecting the dots between you and your partner.

- **Listening actively:**

Pay attention to your coworker. It's as if everyone is tuned in to the same frequency, ensuring comprehension.

- **Spending Quality Time:**

Spend time together. It's like tending to the roots of your superhero romance.

Pleasure-Focused Practices:

● Massages that are sensual:

Look into sensual massages. It's like using touch to create a bonding experience.

Mutual Investigation:

Look into each other's desires. It's similar to discovering hidden treasures in a superhero adventure.

● Laughing Aloud:

Intimate moments can bring you joy. It's like injecting some levity into your conversation.

Finally, sexual health revitalization entails embracing change and discovering new ways for your superhero relationship to thrive. Navigate difficult situations, rediscover intimacy, and investigate holistic approaches.

Your superhero kit includes pelvic floor exercises, communication, and pleasure-focused practices. Remember that it is not about recapturing the past, but about creating a vibrant and fulfilling present in your intimate journey.

Chapter 11: Menopause and Heart Health

Menopause and Cardiovascular Risks

Understanding the link between menopause and heart health is like figuring out the secret ingredients for a heart superhero.

Increased Risk Factors in Menopause:
Menopause may bring additional concerns, such as increases in cholesterol and blood pressure, both of which have an effect on heart health.

Cardiovascular Health Variations:
Consider cardiovascular health to be like a superhero's shield. Menopause may have an impact on how effectively that shield functions.

The Importance of Preventative Cardiovascular Health Measures

Being proactive about heart health is analogous to arming your superhero heart with the greatest weapons and methods for a strong defence.

Heart-Healthy Way of Life

Let's look at several lifestyle choices that may act as a superhero sidekick for your heart, promoting its health and vitality.

Mediterranean Diet and Its Benefits: Diet, Exercise, and Stress Management for Cardiovascular Well-Being

The Mediterranean diet is a meal of superfoods for a healthy heart, including olive oil, fruits, vegetables, and complete grains.

Cardiovascular Workouts for Menopausal Women:

Cardio activities are similar to workouts tailored just for your heart muscle. They maintain their strength and resilience.

Techniques for Stress Reduction for Heart Health:

Stress reduction treatments are like heart-calming spells. They contribute to the maintenance of a tranquil rhythm.

Let's take it a step further:

The Mediterranean Diet and Its Advantages

● Oil of Olives:

In your cooking, use olive oil. It's like arming your heart with a shield of protection.

● Veggies and fruits:

Consume an abundance of fruits and vegetables. They provide nutritional backup.

- **Complete Grains:**

Opt for whole grains. They're like the basis of a superhero with a strong heart.

Walking is a great cardiovascular exercise for menopausal women.

- **Go for vigorous walks**: It's a heart-warming experience that keeps your heroic heart pumping.

- **Swimming:**

Swimming is a good kind of exercise. It's a delicate but powerful splash of delight for your heart.

- **Dancing**:

Listen to your favourite music and dance. It's almost like a hearty celebration of movement.

Techniques for Stress Reduction for Heart Health:

●Breathing deeply:

Deep breathing is recommended. It's like a cool wind for your heroic heart.

● Mindfulness:

Stay in the current moment. It acts as a mental barrier against stress.

● Hobbies and leisure activities:

Take up pastimes that will help you relax. It's a recharge period for your heart superhero.

Finally, menopause and heart health are like travelling buddies on a superhuman quest. Recognize the hazards, take preventative actions, and develop heart-healthy lifestyle behaviours. The Mediterranean diet, customised workouts, and stress-reduction strategies are not simply options; they are tools that will equip your cardiac superhero for a robust and resilient trip through menopause and beyond.

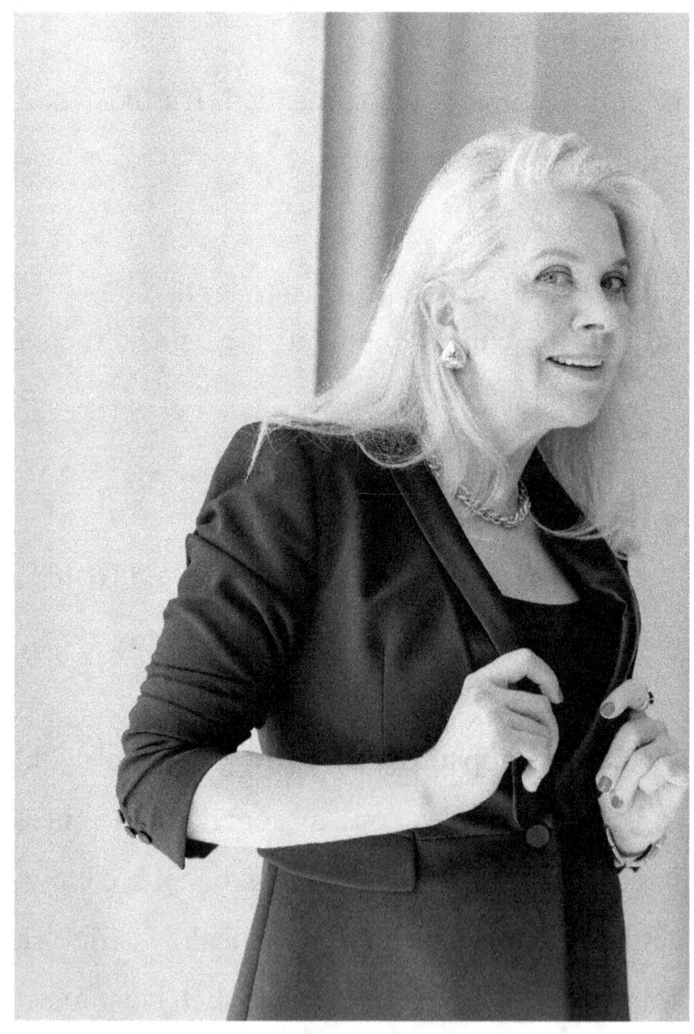

Chapter 12: Comprehensive Approaches to Bone Health

Menopause Bone Health

Understanding bone health during menopause is like uncovering the secret formula for creating a strong and robust bone superhero.

Hormonal Changes and Osteoporosis Risks:

Menopause may be compared to a building site, with hormonal changes influencing how strong the bone structure is created.

Identifying Osteoporosis Risks:

It's like being a detective, searching for evidence that might suggest a risk of osteoporosis, such as a family history or particular drugs.

Early Warning Signs

Early indications of osteoporosis are similar to warning indicators. It's time to take notice if your bones feel weaker or your height decreases.

Developing Strong Bones

Consider strengthening strong bones as constructing a superhero stronghold, where every brick counts for a powerful framework.

Nutrition, Exercise, and Lifestyle for Bone Density

Let's look at the tools and tactics for fortifying your bone superhero and creating a castle that stands tall and powerful.

Calcium-Rich Foods and Supplements

● Calcium-Rich Foods:

Calcium-rich meals, including milk, cheese, yoghurt, and leafy greens, act as building elements for your bone heroes.

● Supplements:

Supplements are like reinforcements for your superhero stronghold. Calcium supplements may help if food alone isn't adequate.

Weight-Bearing Exercises for Bone Strength Walking:

Walking is similar to giving your bones a daily workout. It is mild yet helpful in increasing bone strength.

● Dancing:

Dancing is like a vibrant party for your bones. It mixes movement with weight-bearing, which strengthens bones.

- **Strength Training:**

Strength training is similar to lifting weights for your bone superhero. It increases muscular mass, which promotes bone density.

- **Sunlight Exposure:**

Sunlight is a natural superhero power-up. It aids your body's production of vitamin D, which is required for calcium absorption.

- **Healthy Eating Habits**:

A nutritious diet is like superhero fuel for your whole body, especially your bones. It contains a variety of minerals, including vitamin K, magnesium, and phosphorus.

Avoiding Smoking and Excessive Alcohol Consumption:

Smoking and excessive alcohol use are villains attempting to damage your bone superhero. Avoiding them helps to preserve bone strength. Let's break it down further:

Calcium-Rich Foods:

● **Dairy and milk:**

These are the key building components for your bone superhero stronghold.

● **Leafy Greens:**

Leafy greens are like secret spies, slipping in and supplying calcium in a different form.

● **Yoghourt**:

Yogurt is the superhero's companion, providing not just calcium but also probiotics for general wellness.

Weight-Bearing   Exercises: Jumping Jacks:

Jumping jacks are like a pleasant exercise for your bones. They incorporate leaping and arm motions that engage numerous muscle groups.

●Hiking:

Hiking is an outdoor excursion for your bones. The different landscape both challenges and strengthens them.

● Yoga:

Yoga is like a mild superhero exercise. It promotes general bone health by improving balance and flexibility.

Habits of Life:

● Sun exposure:

Spend time in the sun. It's like providing your bone superhero with the natural sunshine it needs to grow.

● **Leafy Greens**:
Include leafy greens in your diet. They're like nutritional superheroes, providing a range of bone-supporting elements.

● **Moderation in Alcohol:**
If you love alcohol, drink it in moderation. It's like striking the correct balance to keep your bone superhero castle strong.

To summarise, holistic bone health in menopause is much more than simply calcium. Understand the dangers, ingest a range of nutrients, participate in weight-bearing workouts, and adopt lifestyle practices that promote bone strength. Building strong bones is similar to creating a superhero castle that is durable and defends your general well-being.

Chapter 13: Exiting the Menopause Reset Code

Reflections on the Journey

Let's take a minute to reflect on the menopausal journey—it's like looking back at a map and realising how far you've come.

Recognizing and Celebrating Achievements:

Celebrate minor successes. It's similar to earning badges on your menopausal journey.

Managing Menopausal Changes:

Managing changes is like piloting a ship through unfamiliar seas. Each modification is a step toward smoother sailing.

Personal Development Self-Reflection:

Personal development is like the superhero cape you've earned. Accept the modifications and examine your progress.

Resilience:

Resilience is the superhuman force inside you. It enables you to overcome problems and keep going ahead.

Keeping Hormonal Balance

Consider hormonal harmony to be a song that maintains your body in sync, like a superhero with a harmonic soundtrack.

Long-Term Strategies for Maintaining Well-Being Maintaining Lifestyle Changes:

Lifestyle modifications are like the continuing storyline of your superhero narrative. Continue to practise those routines for hormonal balance.

Ongoing Hormonal Balance:

Ongoing hormonal balance is like a dance, with steps changing as the music of menopause plays on.

Adaptation Techniques:

Changing tactics is similar to having a diverse tool kit. Adapt and adjust as your menopausal requirements change.

Let's break it down further:

Celebrating Success:

● **Daily Winnings:**

Small everyday victories should be celebrated. It's like adding glitz to your menopausal journey.

● **Trying Out New Approaches**:

Trying fresh techniques is like going along various roads. Even if some don't work, it's still progress.

●Seeking Help:

Seeking help is like bringing sidekicks into your menopausal experience. Share your successes with others.

Personal Development Reflection: Learning from Obstacles:

Learning from adversities is similar to acquiring experience points. Each difficulty makes you stronger.

Adapting to Changes:

Adapting to change is like updating your superhero costume. It guarantees that you are prepared for anything that comes your way.

Finding Your Inner Strength:

Finding inner strength is similar to uncovering a secret superpower inside oneself. It was always there; you just needed to realise it.

Maintaining Lifestyle Changes:

• Consistency:

Consistency is like the beat of your heroic music. Maintain your lifestyle adjustments for a harmonic balance.

• Healthy Eating Habits:

Healthy eating habits are like nourishing gasoline for your superhero body. They keep you energetic and lively.

• Regular Exercise:

Regular exercise is similar to the superhero workout plan. It maintains the strength and flexibility required for the voyage.

Adaptation Techniques:

● **Listening to Your Body**:

Pay attention to your body's signals. It's like listening to the music and modifying your steps appropriately.

● **Seeking Professional Advice**:

Seeking expert advice is similar to having a mentor in your superhero training. Experts may give helpful insights.

● **Embracing Change:**

Accepting change is like flipping the page to the next chapter. It's a continuation of your ongoing menopausal narrative.

Finally, shutting the menopausal reset code is about accepting a continual journey rather than attaining a goal. Recognize progress, praise accomplishments, and reflect on personal improvement. sustaining hormonal harmony entails sustaining lifestyle modifications, achieving continuing balance, and modifying techniques. It's like writing a dynamic superhero story—one that grows and continues to inspire you in the coming chapters.

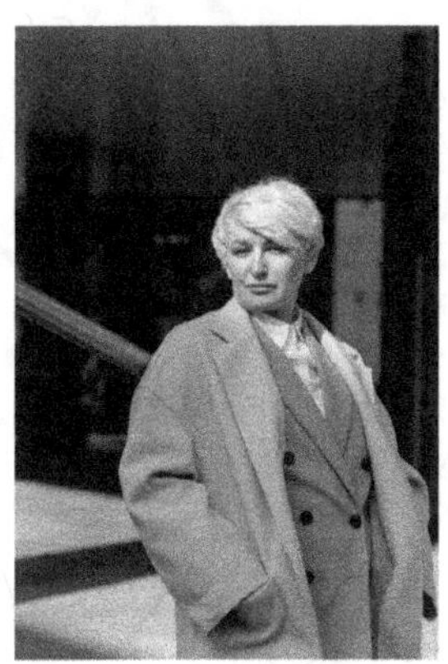

Conclusion: Menopausal Empowerment

Let's summarise our powerful experience through menopause—it's like collecting the spoils of our expedition.

Understanding Changes: A Recap of Key Insights and Strategies

We discovered that menopause brings about changes, much like a superhero emerging with new abilities.

Holistic Methodologies:

Nutrition, exercise, and a healthy lifestyle are our superhero weapons for living a balanced existence.

Honouring Achievements:

In our menopausal journey, celebrating accomplishments, large or little, is like collecting trophies.

Changing Situations:

Adapting to changes is analogous to altering our superhero capes to tackle each twist and turn.

Encouragement for Embracing Menopause with Vitality Embracing Wisdom:

The postmenopausal period is like unleashing the knowledge of a superhero. Accept the experience.

Every Chapter Has Life:

Every stage of life is a new adventure. Take it on with the vigour of a superhero.

Developing Resilience:

Building a superhero castle is similar to cultivating resilience. It strengthens and stabilises us.

Passing the Torch: A Call to Action for Sharing the Menopause Reset Code with Others

It's like passing the heroic torch when you share the Menopause Reset Code. Allow others to benefit from your knowledge.

Creating a Community of Support:
A supporting community is like a superhero team. We can empower and encourage one another if we work together.

Menopause Movement Formation:
The Menopause Reset Code is a rallying cry encouraging women to live powerful lives.

Let's take a closer look:

Key Insights and Strategies Recap:

Understanding Transitions:

Menopause is a natural process:

Menopause is a normal stage in a woman's superhuman journey. It's all part of the adventure.

Hormones at Work:

Hormones, like superhero teammates, play a part. Understanding them will assist you in navigating the changes.

Holistic Methodologies:

Nutrition that is well-balanced:

Nutritional balance is analogous to supplying heroic fuel. It maintains our bodies fit and powerful.

Exercise Program:

Workout programs are similar to superhero workouts. They keep our strength and flexibility in check.

Lifestyle Options:

Lifestyle choices are analogous to the superhero code. They point us in the direction of a full and satisfying existence.

Honouring Achievements:

Minor Victories:

Small successes are like everyday superhero missions. It keeps us going.

Trying New Approaches:

Trying new techniques is like adding new tools to our superhero toolbox. It broadens our capacities.

Encouragement to Welcome the Post-Menopausal Period with Vitality:

● Life Advice:

Life after menopause is like having wisdom superpowers. Accept the lessons acquired.

● Navigating Difficulties:

Taking on obstacles is similar to becoming a seasoned superhero. Use the knowledge you've obtained to overcome challenges.

Every Chapter Has Life:

● Positive Prognosis:

In our superhero narrative, a good attitude is like the sun. It adds colour to every chapter.

- **Taking on New Challenges**:

Accepting new challenges is like flipping the page to fresh and exciting possibilities. Each chapter is alive and well.

Learning from Setbacks: Cultivating Resilience:

Learning from failures is similar to increasing our resilience. It guarantees that we recover stronger.

Developing Inner Strength:

Inner strength is the foundation of our superhuman power. It helps us persevere in the face of adversity.

Call to Action for Spreading the Menopause Reset Code:

- **Exchanging Experiences**:

Sharing experiences is like handing out long heroic stories. It bridges generations.

- **Supporting One Another:**

Supporting one another is similar to building a superhero team. We are stronger together.

- **Creating Connections: Creating a Supportive Community:**

Making relationships is like constructing a superhero circle. It gives power via togetherness.

- **Resource Sharing:**

Sharing resources is analogous to assembling a team of superheroes. It guarantees that everyone gets what they need.

- **Empowering Women: Creating a Menopause Movement**

Women's empowerment is akin to sparking a superhero revolution. It changes people's lives.

● **Breaking Down Barriers**:
Breaking down stigmas is like removing roadblocks in our superhero's path. It paves the way for a more promising future.

Finally, our menopause journey is a superhero tale full of insights, strategies, and empowerment. Accept the knowledge you've gained, approach each chapter with vigour, cultivate resilience, and spread the Menopause Reset Code to build a supportive community and a menopause movement. It's more than just the end of a book; it's the start of a new, empowered chapter in your superhero life.